Table of Contents

Obesity Diet

It is a well-known fact that obesity is one of the leading health concerns in today's world, being responsible for more than 325,000 deaths in the United States alone. People who are obese, i.e., those who have a Body Mass Index (BMI) reading of more than 30 are at a very high risk of suffering from various diseases, which include diabetes, heart problems, strokes, high blood pressure and many more. Fortunately, as the awareness of obesity and the problems that are associated with it grows, most of the people who are morbidly overweight have begun taking steps to reach their health weight goal, as soon as possible. Unfortunately, there are many people who resort to obesity diet pills and supplements, which may suppress their appetite and help them lose weight rapidly. However, there are some severe side effects that have been associated with the use of such methods. Others follow a crash diet for reducing weight, which may also help in getting rid of the extra pounds quite rapidly; however, the diets could lead to nutritional deficiencies if continued on a long term basis and once discontinued, people are likely to gain more weight than they had lost. Therefore, it may be best for people to follow a proper, healthy obesity diet and exercise plan instead, which can help them lose weight at a moderate, but steady pace. Since obesity in children is also one of the biggest concerns faced by most parents, it is important for them to seek help and design a healthy childhood obesity diet. An effective and nutritious obesity diet plan not only allows people to reach their weight goal at a fast pace, it also improves their overall health, by increasing energy and boosting their immunity.

In case of people who have a BMI of more than 35, the best option may be to undergo a bariatric weight loss surgery. However, people who have a BMI between 30 and 35 may be able to reach their healthy weight range by following a healthy diet for obesity, a good workout routine and making a few healthy lifestyle changes. For maximum effectiveness, people should plan an obesity diet chart, which includes a wide variety of nutritious foods that have been prepared using healthy cooking techniques. The first step is to identify how many calories are being consumed on a daily basis and then check with a nutritionist about how many calories should be consumed each day, based on factors like gender, age, height, weight and levels of physical activity. Some of the suggestions of a healthy diet chart to reduce weight are to eliminate calories that come from sugar or oil and to reduce portions consumed at each meal.

Most people are under the impression that when following an obesity menu, they will end up consuming bland, boring and tasteless meals on a daily basis. However, this is not true at all, as several obesity diet recipes that enable people to consume their favorite food, prepared in a healthy manner, flavored with healthy spices and herbs. Moreover, a diet in obesity allows people to eat a wide variety of foods, which include fresh fruit, vegetables, fish, skinless poultry, whole grains, certain cereals, seeds and low fat dairy products. Such a diet meets the obesity dietary needs of most people, eliminating unhealthy foods like saturated fats and trans-fats from a diet. To control obesity, diet soda too, must be eliminated from your diet.

Obesity Diet Menu

Given below is a sample of a menu for obese people, based on obesity diet recommendations:

• Early morning: Warm water with the some freshly squeezed lemon juice

• Breakfast: Wheat or chickpea sprouts, with a cup of skim milk

- Morning Snack: Carrot juice of orange juice

- Lunch: Garden Salad or a mixture of steamed veggies, like cucumber, carrots, cauliflower, beetroot, onions and tomatoes

- Evening Snack: Vegetable soup or coconut water

- Dinner: Steamed Salmon, with half a cup of brown rice and half an orange

It is important for people to realize that obesity dietary management is a long term commitment, more like a lifestyle change, which needs to be followed on a continual basis. There are numerous obesity dietary guidelines that are easily available through online resources and health articles. However, it is absolutely essential to check with a doctor and get an approval, before following any of these guidelines.

Obesity Food

Following an obesity meal plan usually enables people to lose their excess pounds and reach their healthy weight as soon as possible. It is a well-known fact that obesity foods to avoid include fried food, junk food, sugar, processed food, as well as those food items that are calorie dense or high in starch. However, while people may be aware of the foods that should be avoided when following a weight loss diet plan, not a lot of people are aware of what the healthy obesity foods to eat are.

Food for reducing weight

Given below are some of the healthy foods that should be incorporated in a weight loss diet:

• Between 4 to 7 servings of fresh fruits and vegetables each day, as they are loaded with vitamins, minerals, fiber and antioxidants. These foods are not just good for weight loss, but also reduce risks of diseases

• Whole grains like whole wheat bread and pasta, breakfast cereal (low sugar), brown rice, buckwheat, quinoa, barley, oat bran and oats.

• Low fat dairy products such as skim milk, plain yogurt and cottage cheese

• Seeds and a few varieties of nuts

• High quality protein, which is low in fat, like chicken, turkey, legumes and fish

Many obese people are advised to follow a juice diet or the juice fast for a period of a week or so, so that they can shed the excess extra pounds faster. Health and nutrition experts advise people to consume fresh fruit or vegetable juice for obesity.

Before following any diet plan or making any major changes to an existing diet, it is important to consult a doctor and get an approval. This is all the more important for people who are elderly or are suffering from any preexisting medical condition. Pregnant women too, should be careful before following any diet plan and should consult a doctor before doing so.

Diet Plan for Obesity

Obesity is a condition resulting from accumulation of excess body fat and this is becoming a major health concern which increases the risk of several other Health issues.It is evaluated by body mass Index and If BMI is 30 or higher than thirty then the person is obese .Low fat, low carbohydrates and moderate protein diet is very helpful in loss of excess fat.

The diseases caused by obesity include Diabetes, Heart disease, Arthritis, Cancer, liver problems, infertility and many more.Body weight has to be maintained to diminish the risk of these diseases and which is only possible with proper healthy diet.

DIET CHART FOR OBESITY

EARLY-MORNING

Indian gooseberries -3-4 (cooked) / Aloe Vera juice- 20 ml

BREAKFAST

Broken Wheat Porridge (Veg dalia) / Veg Semolina (veg upma) /oatmeal/ Veg Vermicelli (Sewian) / Stuffed Chapatti / Chapatti with veg or dal/Beetroot Juice / Pomegranate Juice

MID-MORNING

Fruit/ Green juice / Coconut water

LUNCH

Plain chapatti / Multi grain chapatti / Boiled Brown Rice / Veg khichdi/ Vegetable + Dal + Salad

EVENING

Herbal Tea / Red juice / Sprouts / Fox nuts/ Roasted chickpea/ Granola bar (Homemade)

DINNER

Plain chapatti / Boiled Rice / Khichdi / Dalia / Sabudanakhichdi/ Vegetable + Dal + Salad

DIET INSTRUCTIONS

CEREALS

Cereals to be consumed

Wheat, Brown rice, Brown bread, Oatmeal, Quinoa, Barley, Pulses

Cereals to be avoided

White rice, White flour, White bread, Pasta

FRUITS

Fruits to be consumed

Black currant, Peach, Apple, Pear, Papaya, Orange, Lemon, Guava, Kiwi, Pomegranate,

Fruits to be avoided

Mango, Banana,Litchi

VEGETABLES

Vegetables to be consumed

Green leafy vegetables like Spinach, Green onions, Carrots, Beetroots, Tomatoes,Radish, Okra, Cabbage, Broccoli, Cauliflower, Mushroom, Zucchini, Pumpkin, Beans, Cucumber, Garlic, Ginger.

Vegetables to be avoided

Potatoes, Sweet potato

PULSES

Pulses to be consumed

Green gram, Redlentil, pigeon pea, Kidney beans, black beans and mostly lentils are good for obesity

Pulses to be avoided

Black gram, dried and frozen pulses

DAIRY PRODUCTS

Dairy Products to be consumed

Skimmed milk, Buttermilk, Cottage cheese

Dairy Products to be avoided

Butter, Cheese, coconut milk

SPICES

Spices to be consumed

Fenugreek, Pepper, Cloves, Mint, Turmeric, Cinnamon, Mustard, Coriander, Parsley

Spices to be avoided

Nil

DRINKS

Drinks to be consumed

Green tea, homemade vegetable juices, coconut water, Herbal tea

Drinks to be avoided

Beverages such as soda, cold drinks, alcohol, Energy drinks, Fruit syrups

FLESH FOODS

Flesh Foods to be consumed

Lean meat chicken, Salmon, Egg white.

Flesh Foods to be avoided

Red meat and Processed meat

SEEDS AND DRY FRUITS

Dry Fruits to be consumed

Pumpkin seeds, Chia seeds, Walnuts, Almonds (soaked)

Dry Fruits to be avoided

Sunflower seeds, Cashew, Dates, prune

OILS

Oils to be consumed

Olive oil, Canola oil

Oils to be avoided

Corn Oil, sunflower oil, Rice bran oil, cotton seed oil

OTHER FOODS

Other Foods to be consumed

Sprouted nuts, Sprouts grain

Other Foods to be avoided

Junk food, Coconut cream and milk, Pastries, Puffs, Frozen and simple Yoghurt, Roasted dry fruits, Sugar products.

LIFESTYLE AND DIETARY TIPS

- Do not skip meals. Eat three balanced meals.

- Avoid intake of fatty and sugary food.

- Eat seasonal fruits and vegetables.

- Avoid late night snacking.

- Increase fiber intake.

- Choose low- calorie food.

- Increase physical activities.

- Drink 8- 10 glasses of water daily.

Diet Chart For Obesity Patient

A low fat diet, as the name implies, is a dietary pattern that limits the fat intake at about 1/3 of the total daily calories consumed. It consists of little fat, particularly saturated fats and cholesterol which lead to increased blood cholesterol levels and heart attack.

This type of diet plan to reduce obesity focuses on foods that contain whole grains, fruits and vegetables. It is directed towards weight loss and treatment of certain diseases by offering 20 to 30 percent of total daily calories from fat. Plenty of vegetables and proteins in a typical low fat diet supply the body with energy but very little fats.

However, fats should not be eliminated entirely as some dietary fat is needed for good health, supplying energy and fat soluble vitamins like A, D, E and K. Studies have revealed that the right kinds of fats can actually help in losing weight. Hence, the prime focus of healthy diet plan for obesity is on limiting the unhealthy fats and consumption of right amounts of fats.

Low-fat diets have been promoted for the prevention of heart disease. Lowering fat intake from 35-40% of total calories to 15-20% of total calories has been shown to decrease total and LDL cholesterol by 10 to 20%; however, most of this decrease is due to a reduction in saturated fat intake.

We create an Indian diet chart for people facing obesity. Follow this diet plan and start eating those food items which listed in breakfast, lunch and dinner timings.

1 Week Diet plan for obesity patient

Sunday

Breakfast (8:00-8:30AM): 3 egg whites + 1 toasted brown bread + 1/2 cup low fat milk (no sugar)

Mid-Meal (11:00-11:30AM): 1 cup papaya

Lunch (2:00-2:30PM): 1 cup arhar dal + 1 chapatti + 1/2 cup low fat curd + salad

Evening (4:00-4:30PM): 1 cup vegetable soup

Dinner (8:00-8:30PM): 1 cup pumpkin + 1 chapatti + salad

Monday

Breakfast (8:00-8:30AM): 1 onion stuffed chapatti + 1/2 cup low fat curd

Mid-Meal (11:00-11:30AM): 1 cup coconut water

Lunch (2:00-2:30PM): 1 cup moong dal/ chicken curry + 1 chapatti + salad

Evening (4:00-4:30PM): 1 cup pomegranate

Dinner (8:00-8:30PM): 1 cup beans + 1 chapatti + salad

Tuesday

Breakfast (8:00-8:30AM): 2 besan cheela + 1/2 cup low fat curd

Mid-Meal (11:00-11:30AM): 1 apple

Lunch (2:00-2:30PM): 1 cup masoor dal + 1 chapatti + 1/2 up low fat curd + salad

Evening (4:00-4:30PM): 1 cup tomato soup

Dinner (8:00-8:30PM): 1 cup carrot peas vegetable +1 chapatti + salad

Wednesday

Breakfast (8:00-8:30AM): 1 cup vegetable brown bread upma + 1/2 cup low fat milk (no sugar)

Mid-Meal (11:00-11:30AM): 1 cup musk melon

Lunch (2:00-2:30PM): 1 cup rajma curry + 1 chapatti + salad

Evening (4:00-4:30PM): 1 cup vegetable soup

Dinner (8:00-8:30PM) 1 cup parwal vegetable + 1 chapatti + salad

Thursday

Breakfast (8:00-8:30AM): 1 cucmber hungcurd sandwich + 1/2 tsp green chutney + 1 orange

Mid-Meal (11:00-11:30AM): 1 cup buttermilk

Lunch (2:00-2:30PM): 1 cup white chana/ fish curry + 1 chapatti + salad

Evening (4:00-4:30PM): 1 cup low fat milk (no sugar)

Dinner (8:00-8:30PM): 1 cup cauliflower vegetable + 1 chapatti + salad

Friday

Breakfast (8:00-8:30AM): 1 cup vegetable poha + 1 cup low fat curd

Mid-Meal (11:00-11:30AM): 1 cup watermelon

Lunch (2:00-2:30PM): 1 cup chana dal + 1 chapatti + salad

Evening (4:00-4:30PM): 1 cup sprouts salad

Dinner (8:00-8:30PM): 1 cup tinda vegetable + 1 chapatti + salad

Saturday

Breakfast (8:00-8:30AM): 1 cup low fat milk with oats + 3-4 strawberries

Mid-Meal (11:00-11:30AM): 1 cup coconut water

Lunch (2:00-2:30PM): 1 cup soybean curry + 1 chapatti + 1/2 cup low fat curd + salad

Evening (4:00-4:30PM): 1 cup fruit salad

Dinner (8:00-8:30PM): 1 cup ghia vegetable + 1 chaptti + salad

Do's And Dont's While following Diet Plan for Obesity

Try to avoid these food items if you are following obesity diet plan:

1. Rely on soft drinks, sweetened cereals, cookies and cakes, donuts and pastries, chips, and confectionery to get you through the day.

2. Don't skip meals. This will tempt you to snack and DO NOT snack between meals

3. Avoid eating quickly. Sit and chew each bite. Try using chopsticks!

4. Don't food shop when you're hungry.

5. Don't eat more than two or three pieces of fruit per day

Add these food items if your diet chart if you are following obesity diet plan :

1. Eat more vegetables - add them at every meal.

2. Drink plenty of water - you can become hungry when thirsty.

3. Try eating off smaller plates so as to eat smaller portions

4. Exercise between 30 minutes to one hour each day with moderate exercise - brisk walking, team sport, cycling or swimming.

5. Be mindful of what you put in your mouth and your shopping trolley.

Food Items You Can Easily Consume In Obesity Diet Plan

1. Choose minimally processed, whole foods:

2. Whole grains (whole wheat, steel cut oats, brown rice, quinoa)

3. Vegetables (a colorful variety-not potatoes)

4. Whole fruits (not fruit juices)

5. Nuts, seeds, beans, and other healthful sources of protein (fish and poultry)

6. Plant oils (olive and other vegetable oils)

7. Drink water or other beverages that are naturally calorie-free

www.ingramcontent.com/pod-product-compliance
Lightning Source LLC
Chambersburg PA
CBHW060923130726

48001CB00006B/2381